As with any change in eating and/or exercise, I advise you to get a complete medical evaluation. Being a chiropractor, I also recommend getting a complete chiropractic evaluation. The statements made in this book have not been evaluated by the Food and Drug Administration (U.S.). Nothing in the following pages is intended to diagnose, treat, cure or prevent any condition or disease. Again, please consult with your own medical or osteopathic physician or other medical specialist regarding the suggestions and recommendations.

As with any eating or exercise plan, there are risks and benefits. It is up to you and your physician to determine the risk/benefit ratio. Below is an incomplete list of benefits and risks. Again, please consult with your medical professional to determine what is best for you.

 Benefits: Participation in a regular program of physical activity has been shown to produce positive changes. These changes include increased work capacity, improved cardiovascular efficiency, and increased muscular strength, flexibility, power, and endurance. Additionally, studies have shown following a controlled-carbohydrate diet provides benefits to your health, including weight loss.

Risks: You realize that exercise and dietary changes can carry some risk to the musculo-skeletal system (strains, sprains) and the cardio-respiratory system (dizziness, discomfort in breathing, heart attack). You hereby certify that you know of no medical problem that would increase your risk of illness and injury because of participation in a regular exercise program. Additionally, your decision to begin a diet and exercise program is yours alone and Joe Leonardi will not be liable for damages arising out of or in connection with the use of the information provided in this book.

Results may vary and are not guaranteed.

Prologue

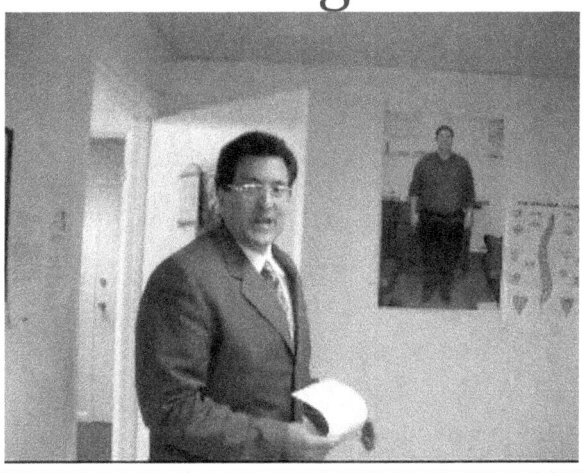

Recidivism – From Merriam-Webster: a tendency to **RELAPSE** into a previous condition or mode of behavior.

The following is about my battle with obesity recidivism, my methodology and my lifestyle. What you read may offend, although I hope not. I have turned over a new leaf in my life, while I may disagree with others, I will not run down another person because I may disagree with their theories and methodology.

With that said, I will never lose my hard edge, honesty or belief in self-responsibility and self-accountability when it comes to battling obesity and improving our fitness.

It is my intent and hope, that by sharing my battle with recidivism, that I may inspire you, the reader, not to give up, not to quit and most importantly — know that you aren't alone in this battle. Together, once we identify the causes and problems, we can then overcome the bastard that is obesity.

Aloha, Ciao and Stay Healthy,

Joe

Introduction

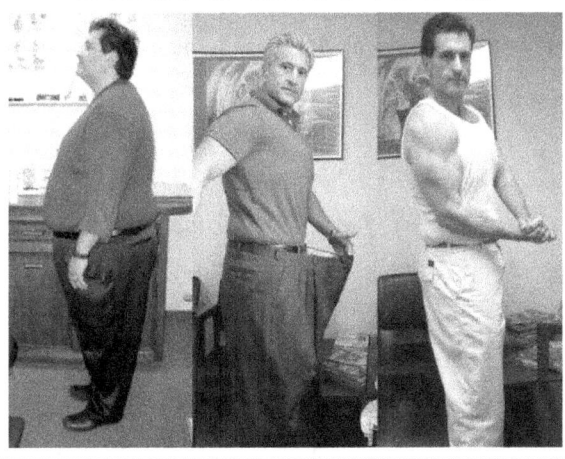

My name is Joe Leonardi, that is me in the above photo's, all three pictures. The first image was me at 340lbs, in March of 2008. The other two I go somewhere around 210lbs, and yes I went blonde for a little while — I think once I knock this bout of recidivism on its ass, I may go back to the light colored locks.

I am a chiropractor and for the last three and half years, I **was** a physical culturist. I had dropped over one hundred and thirty pounds in about a year and kept it off for more than three. I wrote a book about my experience and I gave over forty interviews on the topics of weight loss, fitness, obesity, childhood obesity and bullying. In my mid-forties, I was in the best shape of my life since I was in my early twenties. I ate a healthy, low carbohydrate, natural diet, did some type of exercise seven days a week and kept a high energy, positive outlook on life.

Then, I backslid, not all the way back to 340 pounds, but far enough. The picture on the cover is from July of 2013, that was when I finally woke up. How far did I backslide? Too far!

This short book is my journey back from the depths of recidivism forward — returning to a lifestyle focused on health, wellness and fitness. I will tackle what I like to call the 5 deadly sins of obesity relapse, the 5 stages of weight re-gain and finally, 5 myths of weight loss — of course, all from my point of view.

There is one person responsible for my backslide and one person alone — that is the guy I see in the mirror every morning. I had some stressful times, but we all have stress. Stress and pressure are something that must be dealt with on a daily basis. Most of those stressors I had absolutely no control over, however, I did have control over how I chose to respond — I chose poorly.

I allowed myself to fall back into old patterns of eating a junk food laden diet. As the nutrient deficient food robbed my body of its strength and vitality — exercising became a less desirable activity. Eventually, the ability to sleep through the night became impossible and most days started off hazy and harried, zipping through fast food drive through after fast food drive through for overly processed, carbohydrate loaded, energy dense/nutrient devoid trash. Those food *stuffs* became my sustenance of choice. As my eating and exercise faltered, my mental energy plummeted to the depths of pessimism. I tuned into local talk radio just to hear others bound together by the common bond of despair. Positive attitudes were replaced by negative acceptance — and further into the void my health, fitness and wellness sunk.

I was ready to give up and give in — to be done with eating healthy, exercising regularly and staying positive. It was time to embrace the demons of doom, and no longer promote nor advocate for the life I had lived so happily for the previous three and a half years. I even wrote about it. The below posting is as it appeared on my blog. It was an honest assessment of my recidivism and my failed attempt to get back on track. If you are reading this book, then it means I have gotten back on track, and I am once again on my way to being fit and healthy.

An Important Week

Today is Tuesday, July 16, 2013.

This is the most important week of my life.

As most of you know, I have been having a very difficult time getting back to eating a healthful diet and following a fitness encouraging exercise program.

My mental energy has been at an all-time low — I didn't recover from what happened last year. Amazingly, it was something I never thought could happen to me. It seems so miniscule, but it had an impact on me; and I still haven't been able to will myself past it.

Therefore, I have made an important decision.

If I don't succeed in getting back on track this week — I am done.

No more interviews.

No more fitness and weight loss postings or videos.

And, most importantly, no more claim to being a physical culturist.

If I don't succeed on getting back on track this week — I am done.

I will accept the permanency of my failure; embrace the sloth and gluttony that has once again overtaken me, and I will fade away from the low carb, paleo, primal and fitness worlds. I will delete my websites, blogs, YouTube pages, remove my book from circulation and simply go gentle into that good night.

Reading those words once again, I can say they are what inspired me — I am back and I am ready to not only help people undo their obesity, but battle back the bastard that is recidivism.

What is written here may very well offend or insult some of you — I make no apologies. This book is my experience and my lessons learned. My conclusions are based upon my education, knowledge and my abilities as a clinician to apply that knowledge. If you are one of those who gets offended or insulted, you may not benefit from what I am going to share.

However, if you can get past those feelings, you may garner some useful information from my errors and conclusions and gain some assistance along your way to leading a healthful and more fit lifestyle.

Is Obesity A Disease?

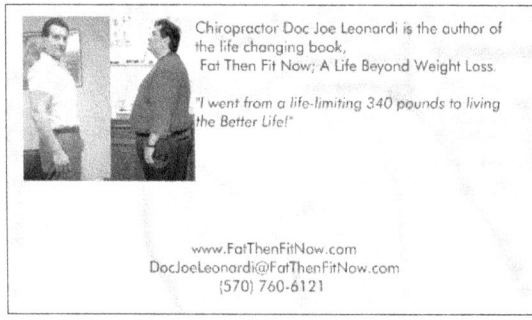

Chiropractor Doc Joe Leonardi is the author of the life changing book,
Fat Then Fit Now; A Life Beyond Weight Loss.

"I went from a life-limiting 340 pounds to living the Better Life!"

www.FatThenFitNow.com
DocJoeLeonardi@FatThenFitNow.com
(570) 760-6121

There is a move to classify obesity as a disease. At the time you are reading this, that may have already occurred. In my opinion, obesity is not a disease. It can be the end outcome of a disease process, and disease can most definitely be the end consequence of obesity — however, unto itself, in the absence of any medical, hormonal, metabolic, etc... underlying cause — obesity is **not** a disease.

Obesity is a physical manifestation. Much like a gas, liquid or solid — the obese body is a physical state of human matter, and as some objects can transcend all three states, it is possible for us to control our bodies, and morph from thin to fit to fat to obese to morbidly obese and back again.

I understand the lure of classifying obesity as a disease. As a healthcare provider, it will allow insurance reimbursement.

Although I don't take insurance in my practice, I can definitely understand how profitable it will be for other healthcare providers to receive reimbursement for their time and services. Then there are those who are overweight, obese, or morbidly obese — ah yes, for the afflicted, it will become the ultimate excuse for not taking responsibility. I can just hear it now; *"It isn't my fault I am overweight — obesity is a disease and dam it I have a condition!"*

In reality, for <u>many</u> of us, it comes down to not wanting to take responsibility and making healthy choices in both diet and exercise.

I am battling back from recidivism. It is a position many of us are familiar with — for whatever reason, those of us who gain weight easily, have a lifetime war with keeping the bastard obesity in check. Yet, no matter the reason, the choices that lead us back up and down are ours — **and no one is going to take that away from me.** I will not allow the excuse makers to take away my self-responsibility or choices.

Much of my attitude about self-responsibility for my own health is shaped by Bernarr MacFadden, Charles Atlas and Jack LaLanne.

These men, in different ways, tried to warn of the impending epidemic that bad choices can lead to and sadly, our current national and global obesity epidemic seems to have proven that they were correct.

I understand the need to blame something or someone, God knows I have wanted to for years. However, in the end, my initial obesity and my recidivism come down to one cause — **giving into weakness.**

I maintained a healthy and fit lifestyle for more than three years. I did it eating an as close to nature low carbohydrate diet and getting in some type of exercise 7 days a week. I was healthy, not as wealthy as I would like, and I guess wise depends on your particular viewpoint. But, the fact that I was healthy cannot be disputed.

The standard medical objective criteria were as close to perfect as possible. My cardiovascular health was fantastic. EKG, echo-cardiogram, stress test were all good, resting heart rate was 54 beats per minute and blood pressure was 110/65. Before that, when I weighed 340 pounds, those criteria were not so good. On my last exercise stress test it took me over 20 minutes to get my heart rate up into the necessary range, during the first one it took about 3, my blood pressure was 140/90 and resting heart rate hung out at just over 90 beats per minute.

While I won't apologize for my opinion, my heart sincerely goes out to those who have a genuine medical condition — those individuals need appropriate medical treatment. For those who can't accept the mantra expressed by Bernarr MacFadden, Charles Atlas, Jack LaLanne and yes, me too — if some medical option will help you get to your goals, who am I to say you are wrong. As state in the header of my blog www.fatthenfitnow.wordpress.com . *"Just remember, even if we disagree, I don't require you to be wrong, for me to be correct in my thinking!"*

Only We Can Decide

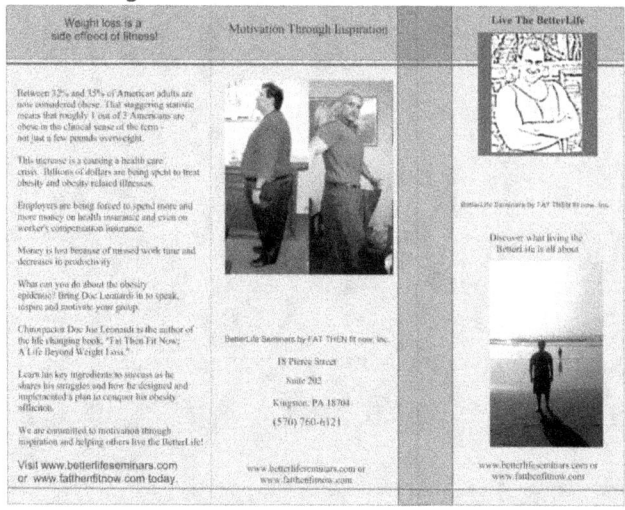

For all that I write or have said, I never tell anyone that he or she must lose weight or get in shape — with one exception, myself.

I have had people ask me if I thought they needed to lose weight and my answer is the same — No. Whether they are 150lbs or 400lbs, it isn't for me to decide who needs to lose weight.

I repeat, it simply isn't up to me.

Yet, they persist, so finally I answer their question with a question. *"Do you think you need to lose weight?"* Their answer will determine if I can assist them.

If they stammer, or have difficulty with an answer — they **aren't** ready.

If they answer, "Yes, I need to lose weight and/or get in shape," — they **might** be ready.

If they answer, "It doesn't matter, I want to lose weight and/or get fit," — they **are** ready.

When it comes to battling obesity and getting fit, we are often looking for external motivation. On occasion, we are seeking validation that we don't need to take control of our health and wellness. Both are irrelevant.

If we want to lose weight — we **must want** to lose weight.

If we want to get fit — we **must want** to get fit.

If we are healthy and fit, can we live a better life? Most definitely, but as it is with everything in life — we must **want** it.

I'm not talking about wanting it, as I want a Ferrari, or a mansion or a beach house. Those are dreams, and many obese people often dream of being fit. No, that kind of wanting never leads to results.

We **must thirst** for it as if we haven't had water in days.

We **must hunger** for it as if we haven't eaten in weeks.

We **must desire** it more than we have ever desired anything in our lives.

However, desire itself isn't enough — that desire must be combined with determination and discipline. To put forth the effort to successfully battle obesity is not for the faint of heart. It genuinely isn't all that difficult, but it does require work and effort. No one is going to pass a wand and make us fit. No one is going to cast a spell and make the fat shed from our bodies.

We must be willing to do the work. We must change our lifestyle to make this happen. A half-hearted, half-assed approach will yield nothing! We must take charge of ourselves and make the necessary changes — we must get moving and we must stop eating health robbing foods and we must have strong and unwavering belief in ourselves.

We must want it with a passion that is second to none, because if we do — only then we will succeed.

Carbohydrate Addiction?

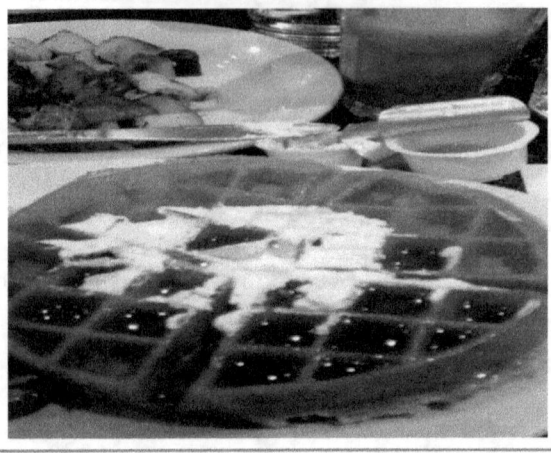

I understand that there are studies that support carbohydrate and sugar addiction, and I also am cognizant of studies that don't support that conclusion — I don't care either way, what I can tell you is one very simple fact:

I am a carb addict.

In my case, it isn't solely sugar, or the simpler carbohydrates, I am addicted to all of them. When I go off the deep end, I just don't have a smattering — I am a full-fledged eating machine.

For three and a half years, I had my carb-addiction under control. Now, I am not a psychiatrist or a psychologist, hell I didn't even stay at a Holiday Inn Express last night, but I do not believe people actually are ever cured of addiction. It is my conviction, from personal experience and observation, that most people swap one dependency for another. Hopefully, we redirect from a negative, sometimes self-destructive, habit to one that is, if not healthier, at least less damaging. For me, the activities I used for redirection were, and are once again, exercising and writing.

The return to carb-cramming didn't occur in one big event, and it wasn't the result of the planned splurges I outlined in my book, Obesity Undone. Funny thing about those planned splurges, when I am mentally geared up and follow precise, meticulous preparation — those carb-meals never bring back the addiction. Why? Because of that planning, I am the one in control of the addiction, not the other way around.

What happened to me developed slowly, over a period of several months. I am sharing this story not for pity, nor sorrow, but to provide an example that it can happen — no matter how much we are convinced it cannot. Also, to demonstrate that if we fall victim to our addiction, we should not quit, give up or cave in — never let the bastard win.

It started in the summer of 2012. It was a dark and stormy night, a shot rang out… Sorry, I love Snoopy….

It did start in the summer of 2012, and it was definitely not the summer of love. I decided to take on some added responsibilities at an institution where I had been working part time. I was expecting to put in a few hours a week, as the duties were explained to me, it should have been a breeze. Well, that summer, to fulfill those extra tasks, I ended up having to take a considerable amount of unplanned time away from my office. That time away hurt my practice, and ended up putting me behind in much of my business work.

The stress was mounting, yet didn't really get to me, but the demands on my time did, and I fell into the fast food habit — but I stayed low carb. However, my attempts to eat as close to nature as possible were getting less close. I was able to stay focused, because no matter the time constraints, I was getting in my daily workout, and being fit caused my body to crave healthful foods to nourish it. Yet, one day in September, it all began to crumble.

I was just finishing up my morning weight training at the gym, when one of the higher ups at my part time employment verbally assailed me over a matter which I had no idea was an issue. I don't mind professionally being taken to task over anything, however this was anything but professional, and in all my adult life, I can't recall being spoken to in such a demeaning manner. To make matters worse, it happened in front of a crowd of people, several of whom happened to be patients. Now, in the old days, before my illness and when my financial situation was much stronger, I would probably have handled it differently. Yet, the reality was, I needed every dime I was earning, additionally, I was just so shocked, that I simply nodded my head and skulked away.

Since I was fourteen years old, whether fat or fit, the gym has been my safe haven. It was, and is, a place I could go to shut out the world and immerse myself in the pleasure of pitting myself against cold, unyielding iron.

Now, perhaps I was just being silly, but the next day, I arrived at the gym and could not bring myself to go in. I was unsure if there would be another unprofessional verbal assault, and of greater concern, I wasn't sure if I could again hold my tongue. Unable to risk my situation, I returned home and showered — then it happened, the insecurities of a bullied youth came rushing to the forefront. And, in my youth, the one response that had brought me through many of the bad times, was to indulge in certain, soothing foods. I went to my favorite breakfast spot and ordered three Belgium waffles and a side of home fires. The nutrient deficient, carb-crammed garbage brought coziness to my mind — at least temporarily. As soon as I finished the last bite, I had immediate buyer's remorse. This wasn't planned, but I thought I could handle it — and I did, that day. For the next several days, I changed my schedule just enough to avoid contact and get my workouts in — the carb-crisis had seemingly passed. However, I ran into this person again, I was cheerful, putting the incident behind me, starting to believe that I had made much more of it than it was. My cheerful greeting was not returned, and the icy silence I received was a clear indication I had not made more out of it than it was, which to me was, and remains, simple silliness.

If I had bit my tongue with the force that my mind applied, a severe, emergency room visit requiring bleed would have been the end result. I hate to admit to this, but unable to respond, the tormented young boy that I once was, again resurfaced. Immediately, I desired, no I required, the soothing of comfort foods. I repeated my breakfast, but this time, there was no buyer's remorse. The anger and shame were so intense, that a carb-laden breakfast became a carb-loaded lunch which then begat a three day carb-binge, which led to a weekend long carb-induced slumber. Finally, that Monday morning, I was able to get ahold of myself — but it took all the willpower I could muster. Sadly, I avoided the gym.

My time in the gym became less and less frequent, and as my fitness level started to decline, my body started craving different foods. Foods that weren't so nourishing for my overall health and well-being. Every now and then, I would give into those cravings. Unfortunately, the carb-addiction, plus the lack of discipline, along with the negative mental energy that was slowly overtaking my personality, was gaining the upper hand. Therefore, instead of one bad meal, it became two, then a day, and then two and three day — when finally, the addiction had nearly wrestled full control.

As 2012 approached an end, I would have stop and start moments, but I could not get complete mastery over my addiction. 2013 wasn't much better, in fact, the stops became more frequent and of longer duration. By the spring, I was no longer wearing the suits I so loved, and when summer came, the starts became nonexistent and my standard dress became workout shorts and oversized, collared shirts.

Finally, I knew I could no longer let the addiction continue unchallenged — it was then I penned, *"An Important Week."* I gave myself one week to get back on track and if I didn't, there were to be consequences.

I recognized — I had a choice.

I understood — I needed to get the upper hand.

I acknowledged — I must be stronger than the addiction.

If not, the bastard wins, and above all, I don't merely lose, I concede my quality of life.

The Carb Cloud Crested

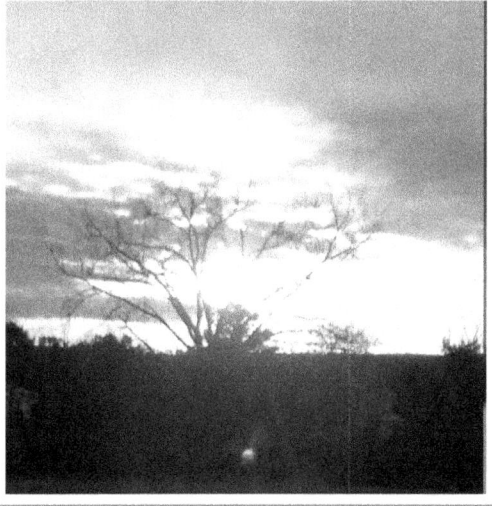

I am back on **my** diet, the diet I had been following faithfully for several years until September 2012, is a diet which is as close to nature as possible and, while I am losing weight, it restricts all starchy carbohydrates. When I am maintaining, I throw in some yams and fruits and on occasion rice or some white potatoes. At the time I am writing this, I have dropped about 48 pounds, so since I still need to shed this remaining God awful layer of lard I added over the last year, my diet does not contain the fruits I enjoy so much.

What's that you ask? Did I use the word diet? Yes, I used the word diet.

But Doc Joe, we aren't supposed to use the "D" word. They say it sets up for failure and makes us feel badly if we don't stick to "a diet."

If you have ever read my book, you know I have very little use for what "they" say. As far as weak-minded bullshit, well I have even less use for — the word is diet! I own it, it is mine and I am not willing to give it up just because "they" the wusses tell me I shouldn't use it. However, I understand that years, hell decades, of misinformation from so-called experts can permeate our thinking. So, just for clarity, I will give my definition of the word.

Diet - anything I put into my gullet and swallow!

Also, when it comes to my diet, I don't care what label one chooses to use; low carb, carb restricted, high protein, high fat, Atkins, Primal, Paleoleithic, Caveman, Ketogenic, JERF and on and on… People get so caught up in the label, they lose sight of what it is all about — eating a healthier diet than the one that we were eating before. Additionally, our diet is not solely or simply about losing weight — it is about living a better and healthier quality of life.

One of the incredible feelings of following a carbohydrate restricted diet is the lifting of **The Carb Cloud**, that brain activity suppressed feeling of being a mental and physical slug. For me, this happened three days into my renewed efforts to recapture my health.

And, the feeling is phenomenal.

One morning, I woke up and my head was clear. It didn't take me as long as it had been taking to start my day. I couldn't wait to get my exercise in. Throughout the day, I didn't find my mind wandering and, no large, loud yawns were escaping my mouth. My energy level was elevated and I found myself not putting routine and mundane tasks off. That evening, I didn't go to bed as early as usual — I simply wasn't tired. Because I was up about three hours later, I thought I would have more difficulty awaking the next morning — but I didn't. For the first time in months, I slept soundly throughout the entire night. So, when the alarm emitted its annoying shriek, I wasn't pulling the covers over my head — however, I must confess, I still wanted to fling the infernal machine against the wall.

It isn't simply the increased energy, which is a huge benefit, but the mental clarity is intoxicating. After eating the standard American trash diet I had been consuming the last few months, all I wanted to do was crawl into a dimly lit corner and crash.

And even when I did take a nap, like the previous evening's sleep, it didn't leave me refreshed as it should — it just left me wanting to doze longer.

I have been asked to explain what I mean when I say; *The Carb Cloud* has vanished by those who haven't experienced this fantastic sensation. It was difficult to put into words, however, a few years back I saw a movie that enabled me to give a very accurate description.   If you have never seen the Bradley Cooper film "Limitless," I highly recommend it, because the scene where Cooper's character takes the mind enhancing drug that activates 100% of his brain — is how it feels when *The Carb Cloud* evaporates.

It is an entirely new outlook on life and the world.

Sin I: Gluttony

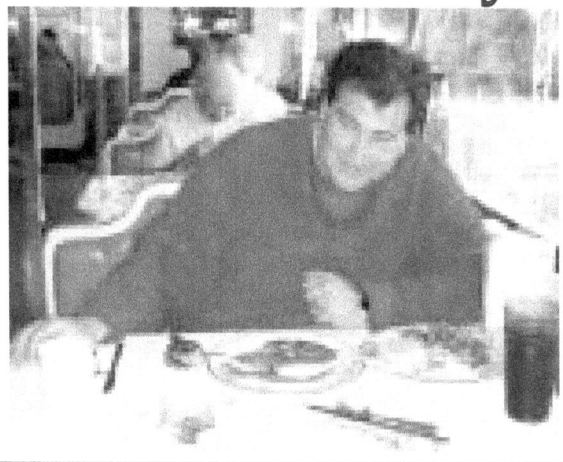

I had gained back a lot of weight! How much exactly? Eighty four pounds, thus moving the pointer on the scale back up to 294!

And let me tell you something — I was, and still am, f*(&ing pissed off.

The summer of last year, that would be 2012 just in case you aren't reading this in 2013, I was in peak physical condition. I weighed in at 210 pounds, I was working out 7 days a week, doing a combination of weight training, sprints, rope skipping and jogging up to 5 miles at a clip and I was eating a healthful, close to nature, low carbohydrate diet.

So, what the hell happened?

Well, for one, I ate too much.

You see, the dirty little secret that all the weight loss gurus, fitness authorities and every other expert doesn't like to talk about, is perhaps one of the biggest truism among the morbidly obese —

I am just going to say it. I know it is going to piss people off, but often times the truth tends to do that.

I AM A GLUTTON!

Yep, I used the *G* word, and when I am done with this book, I am going to use a few other words that those battling obesity don't like too much either. I am going to go even further on this one — it is my opinion, from both observation and helping many people, that most, I said most not all, obese people (the obligatory disclaimer goes here: *If one doesn't have an underlying medical condition*) are gluttons.

I said it.

Yell!

Scream!

Throw your e-reader against the wall — okay don't do that, you won't be able to finish if you are reading an e-book.

Nobody is going to tip the scales at 300, 400, or higher by not eating a whole lot of food. In becoming obese, the issue isn't even what macronutrient is making up the majority of our eating. If we pour pounds upon pounds of porridge down our gullets, we are going to get fat!

Now let's define gluttony. The dictionary definition, from dictionary.com is: *excessive eating and drinking*.

What is excessive? Therein lies the rub. I am going to tell you what excessive was for me.

-Eating so much Goddam food that my pants got tighter while eating. If we have to undo our belts after a meal, we were gluttonous.

-Stuffing so much garbage in my face that I got winded just from chewing. Eating is **NOT** an aerobic activity, we shouldn't be sucking wind just from the simple act of masticating food. If we are, we are gluttonous.

-Engorging myself to the point that the only way I could move is to place both arms on the table for support and lift my massive ass from the chair. Eating isn't supposed to require an expenditure of energy that is so great, that we are actually weakened when the meal is complete.

If you are familiar with these, you too are gluttonous.

I could go on, and I probably will. But the previous three are just simple examples of my gluttony. Go ahead and deny that I haven't described some of you reading this short book. You can deny all you'd like, but the simple fact is that the only person you are being dishonest with, is yourself. God knows, I was.

We must be honest with ourselves. I made every excuse in the past, and unbelievable to me — I fell right back into the same pattern. I was convinced to accept what was supposed to be a part time job, that I should have never taken on. The stress of this part time job, the harassment I was receiving from a higher up when I was trying to work out, yep someone actually had the stones to harass me at the gym where I trained, the drain on my practice, the sucking the life out of my energy and then the dishonesty after I stepped away, all led me back to my path of gluttony.

Boy was I spouting off the excuses — *It was this person's fault for harassing me at the gym, it was that person's fault for not being completely honest with me about what the job entailed, it was this other person's fault for going back on our agreement. Yes, all of those events occurred, but they weren't valid reasons for falling back into gluttony.* I had to be honest with myself, and honest with you, so in turn you can be honest with yourself. If you want the touchy-feely horse crap that has been fed to you time and time again — you aren't going to it here. Excuses and pity and crying and whining and being wussy only lead to giving up on ourselves. I'm going to say something here that may surprise some, you may be think I am being soft — but failure is acceptable. Failure is okay. Failure happens. What isn't acceptable, what isn't okay, what we cannot allow to happen is giving up.

I fell back into the pattern of gluttony because I allowed myself to, I failed and for a time I gave up. But here is the biggest truth — all were my choices. Yes, it was me, myself and I who chose to respond to those stressors by returning to my gluttonous ways.

Food has very calming effects, that is where the term comfort food comes from. At first, I was simply eating more food, and it was still low carbohydrate. Instead of my usual 3 – 4 eggs for breakfast, it began to be 6 or 8. I was adding more cheese to my omelets, having larger portions of steak and even more

and more vegetables. I was eating when I was **NOT** hungry —
and **YES** that is another sign of gluttony.

We eat to energize our bodies, not our minds, not our souls or
any other bullshit reason people claim they need to consume
food. Food is for fuel; nothing more and nothing less. I don't
care what kind of fuel you consume, high fat, high protein, high
carbohydrate, high sugar, high beer… eventually, when you fill
your tank with more fuel than your body needs, the body will
start storing it as body fat. It is much easier to do this with
carbohydrates, that is why low carbohydrates diets are so much
better for weight loss and overall fitness levels. It is beyond
the scope of this book to provide a biochemistry or physiology
course, but when it comes to sugar, if you eat more than you
burn, it converts to fat much easier and more readily than fat or
protein. While I don't adhere 100% to the calories in/calories
out, or eat less/move more mentality — I'm not stupid. The
hell with biochemistry and physiology, common sense will tell
us that excessive amounts of food, even proteins and fats, will
eventually find their way to the spare fuel tank. Anyone who
denies this is a fool. I know — I was one of those people. The
eye opening change in thinking occurred, because even before I
fell away from my healthful diet, I was starting to gain weight,

and even with all the heavy weights I was lifting in the gym, it all wasn't muscle!

So let's call this the spare fuel tank rule; excess fuel if not burned eventually needs to be stored and the lower the quality the fuel, the quicker the conversion to body fat. It has to go somewhere. If you aren't an elite athlete, wait a minute; the hell with elite, because let's face it, most of us aren't athletes, period — we actually have to work for a living. So, if you are a typical American, who works too many hours, sleeps too few hours and your basic idea of exercise is squatting over a public toilet — even if you follow a low carbohydrate diet, you can still eat to excess.

First step — Admit we can be gluttonous.

Second step — Knock it the hell off.

We must be stronger than our weakness. We must understand that we control our choices. We must believe that we can overcome.

What is a good diet to eat? I wrote about that extensively in Obesity Undone and I discuss it on my website www.ObesityUndone.com.

Sin II: Sloth

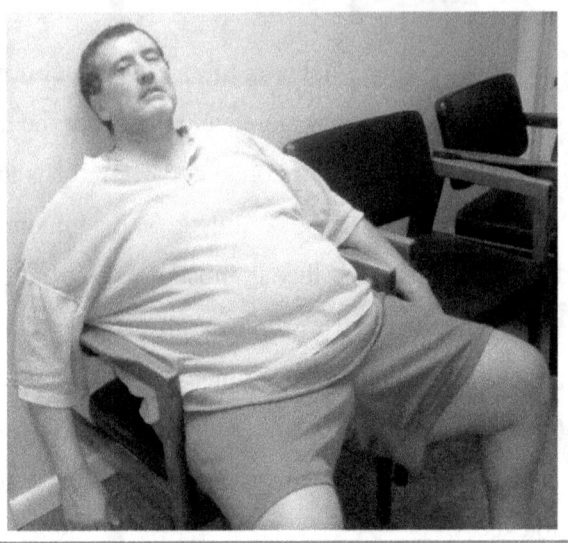

Perhaps the only word more hated by the obese next to gluttony, is sloth. Boy, do we hate that one. I think the reason it gets such a strong reaction is the implication that it means a person is lazy. Well, it doesn't imply that — nope; it comes right out and says it.

Ouch — I just felt a stabbing pain in my right arm. Okay, which one of you has had a voodoo doll of me made up already. Look — I am going to give my view on this particular subject and since the fat ass in the picture is me, photo taken

July 26, 2013, after my obesity relapse, I can confidently say I am an experienced expert on the topic.

As the old question asks, *"What came first?"*

In the case of initial obesity, it is more than likely sloth.

OWWW put down that dam doll!

Look, when I was Joe.340, I have to admit it — I was lazy. Perhaps not in all matters. I mean I did have a full day. Let's take a little peak in a day in the life of Joe.340.

7:00am — Wake up and shower and other morning bathroom activities.

7:30am — Wow, that took some effort, a fifteen minute nap is in order.

7:45am — Wake up again, squeeze into my clothes for the day. Crap, all that effort to suck my gut in was a hell of an ab work out; I need to sit down for a few.

8:15am — I guess that took more out of me than I expected, I fell back to sleep.

8:30am — Breakfast at the local diner. I love diner food. Omelet, short stack of pancakes, home fries, toast and coffee.

Boy that was good, and all this effort to eat and get up out of the chair took some real effort, so I got my work out in.

9:15am — Stop by the local doughnut shop and get the ½ dozen variety back. Then I remembered, I better get another few doughnuts for my staff.

9:45am — Get to the office, thankfully first patients aren't until 10:15, which means I have time for another nap.

Noon — It was a fairly busy morning, thank goodness it is lunch time, but we see patients straight through lunch so I have my office manage order a large pepperoni pizza, fries, and whatever she and the other two chiropractic assistants want.

2:00pm — There is a lull in the action, so I go into my office to catch up paperwork and take 40 winks. I send one of the CA's down to DQ to get us all some ice cream.

6:00pm — We are working through dinner, so we call down to the deli and have a few subs and some chips sent down to the office.

8:00pm — Office is closed and paperwork is done. Stop by local burger place and get three or four burgers and two large orders of fries. The kid at the drive thru asks if I want anything to drink. I get 2 diet cokes, they will go nicely with my favorite whiskey back home.

10:00pm — Fell asleep on the couch, wake up and go to bed.

I know, I know what you're saying, I wasn't lazy — I had a pretty busy day, with all the work between eating an napping.

In Joe.340's case, the sloth definitely led to the obese state. Yes, I worked long hours, and at times the work of a chiropractor can be physical. In those days, I had a very busy practice, but I had periods of sitting on my expanding ass, doing computer work and eating and napping. I was overweight to start with, but I used to workout. The joke at the gym was; here comes Joe, he can lift the gym, but he can't walk around it. The weightlifting kept my weight at about 280lbs, not svelte by any stretch of the imagination, but I did carry around some muscle. But I kind of just stopped going simply because I became lazy and then I got fat(ter).

In this round of recidivism, the answer is definitely the obesity came first. As I discussed in Sin I, the gluttony and my eating pattern evolved from overconsumption of low carb natural foods, to overeating higher and higher and more and more processed junk foods over time. I was still working out, doing my entire workout just as I had been doing the last three plus years, but, sadly, as the weight came on — it became more and more difficult to get my energy level up to workout.

First, I would simply miss part of my workout, usually the jogging or sprints. Then I would sleep a little later, and would have to cut my weight training short. Next, I would miss an entire workout because I was simply too lazy to get in the gym, until eventually, I stopped going altogether. In the recidivism era, obesity led to sloth.

If we don't address the fact that sloth plays a factor in obesity, then we can't address it and do something about it. Sloth is actually easy to beat back — it is purely about discipline.

Discipline in our scheduling.

Discipline in our commitment.

Discipline in making out a plan.

And most importantly, discipline in carrying out that plan.

I am writing this today, 8/12/2013, this is the last day of the first vacation I have had since January of 2011. That vacation I went to California and visited my sister and nephews, this one I stayed here and spent time with my girlfriend and her daughter. In both cases I remained active, but today, I woke up later than usual, which in my case is 7:30am, and I was at my girlfriend's having coffee on the porch sitting with her little Sheltie. It was a beautiful morning, and I didn't want to waste the last day of a vacation apart from "my girls." So, I stayed with them, went out to lunch and just hung around the house. It was a nice day. Would it be just as easy for me to fall back into the pattern of sloth tomorrow? You and I know it would. So, I have already set my alarm clock for 5:00am, I have the coffee in the maker and the timer set and the gym bag and clothes for tomorrow are packed and in the car. It is planning to be disciplined that conquers sloth. It is all about desire, determination and discipline.

When we prepare for our plan, we commit mentally, then we follow through physically — we succeed in winning the war on recidivism.

Don't fear the words, don't fear the realities — face them and face ourselves and victory over the bastard will result.

Sin III: Anger

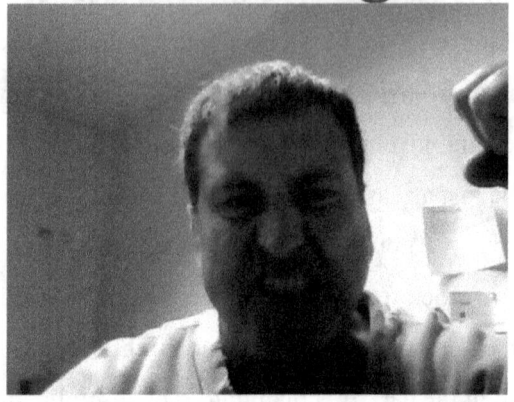

As I stated earlier, I wasn't merely angry, I was pissed off. But who was I angry with? The answer now is easy — I was angry with myself. However, while going through the recidivism, before I woke up and caught it, I was angry at everyone else.

I couldn't lash out, because I guess somewhere deep inside, I was aware that the person to be angry with was this guy named Joe. So, instead of lashing out at those I was "*blaming,*" I externalized my anger through writing and speaking. I keep a blog, Fat Then Fit Now; and through it I brought forth my rage on anyone with whom I even remotely or barely disagreed. I stand by my thoughts, and the sentiments behind much of what I wrote, however I don't care for the way I made things personal.

It is one thing to disagree with others ideas, methods, theories, etc.... and to argue the validity of a point is fine, but when the conversation digress to attacks on the messenger — that is when it is a sure sign of internal anger being redirected at something else. I'm not saying we allow people to walk all over us. I'm not saying we need to back down on our point of view. I'm not saying dishonesty is required. What I am saying is that it is okay to discuss from a diplomatic and professional point of view, and to keep the conversation on the topic and not direct it onto the person with whom we disagree.

I am not the only person in the world to have done this, in psychology they call it displacement. I don't care much for psychological mumbo jumbo, so I will call it what it is — pettiness.

I was angry and that led to me writing stupid things. We don't like to accept blame, but boy o boy do we like to place it. And, that is what I was doing.

Anger is something that needs to be gotten ahold of before we can move forward. Most of us who have engaged in these types of writings and juvenile name calling are really expressing our internal angst outward. Because we aren't in control of ourselves, we go after those with whom we not simply disagree, but in some way we may even envy their success in their chosen discipline or field.

This is easy to do when we are overweight or unfit. There is constant bombardment of the body beautiful and instead of celebrating the success of others, for some reason, many of us attack that success. Maybe it is the entitlement society that we have morphed into. Perhaps it is a sense of envy that many in the academic world pass on in the guise of education to college students by some professors who simply teach, because they could not make it in their chosen field, and teaching is not a passion, but rather a fallback position. Where this act of blaming other actually comes from originates differently for different people, but in this case, the source of the *"blame that person"* mentality isn't that necessary to identify.

It is perfectly fine to simply recognize that we have become one of **those** people, and to overcome that transformation, we simply retrain our brains as we retrain our bodies. We educate ourselves to act kinder, to take a moment before we utter a word, and to not hit the publish or send button for several hours. It is just as easy to be nice as it is to be nasty. It is just as easy to smile as it is to snarl. But when we take a moment to act out of kindness and happiness and joy, we not only make ourselves more positive, we influence those around us with that same positive energy.

Sin IV: Pride's Opposite — Shame

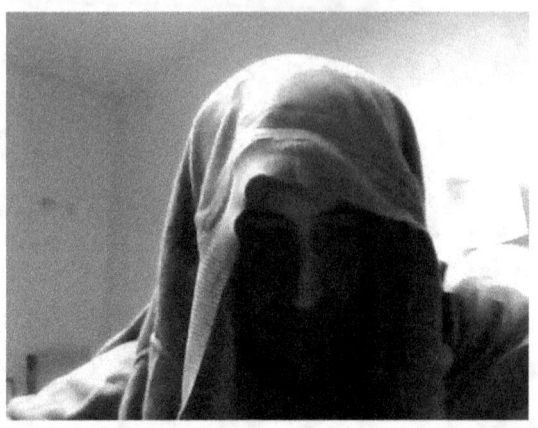

I don't get offended, insulted or embarrassed, but I am a proud person. I have pride in my professions, professionalism and appearance. One of the sad aspects of gaining weight and becoming less and less fit, is that one of my professions, *Physical Culturist*, slowly became null and void. I don't care for hypocrisy, and I avoid it at all costs. It was hard for me to rationalize giving advice on weight loss and fitness as I was gaining weight and becoming not so fit.

Perhaps, most importantly, is my pride in appearance. There is nothing I loathe more than college instructors wearing jeans, untucked shirts and any other clothing that appears less than professional. This summer, I became one of them. Since gaining weight, none of my clothes fit and I was forced to wear shorts and oversized collared shirts. It was, to say the least, humiliating. I thought of purchasing clothing that would fit better, however, then I would be caving into the bastard and who knows, I may never have regained control.

I am hoping my knowledge and concern for my student's education trumped my obviously poor attire. I was given positive feedback from many students, but one of the lessons I like to impart on students is that they should always maintain a professional presence, it was a lesson that I had always tried to teach via example.

I was, and currently, but less so, remain, ashamed of my appearance. For these last several months, this lack of pride stopped me from living life to the fullest. I almost missed going out to Easter brunch with my family, but I was able to squeeze myself into an older, bigger suit. However, I missed many other events and time out. My girlfriend is a saint, she tolerated us not going out much, and becoming homebodies. I never had to tell her, and she never had to ask — but I'm sure she was well aware of why I was retreating into myself.

I know there are those who may think I am overreacting, and perhaps I am, but I would like to share a story that happened a few years ago. It was about six months after my run for congress…. I had just finished up a workout and a walk along the levee. I was dressed in sweats and had on a winter cap. I decided to stop by the grocery store that was adjacent to the levee. Once inside, I ran into an older woman who stopped me and asked me if I was Joe Leonardi. When I told her I was, she had told me she had voted for me. I thanked her. It was then it happened.

She looked me up from head to toe, stood back about a half a step and said, *"I guess you're not going to run again."*

It was my appearance she was commenting on. No matter the reason, I had gone out in public appearing slovenly. At that time it wasn't because of lack of wardrobe, it was just the situation. These days, it is because of giving the bastard the upper hand, and letting myself physically fail.

Sin V: Greed: Yes It Is Good

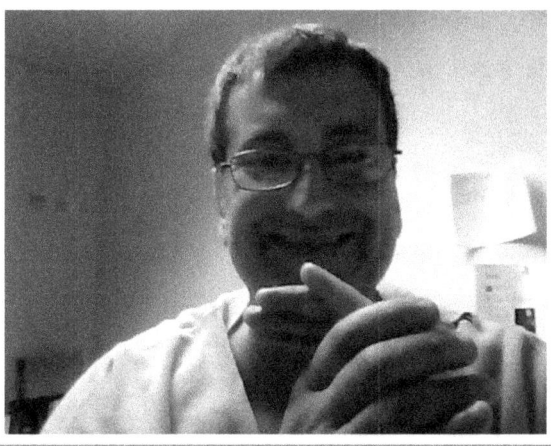

"The point is, ladies and gentleman, that greed, for lack of a better word, is good. Greed is right, greed works. Greed clarifies, cuts through, and captures the essence of the evolutionary spirit. Greed, in all of its forms; greed for life, for money, for love, knowledge has marked the upward surge of mankind." Gordon Gekko; Oliver Stone's Wall Street

For those of us who saw the movie **Wall Street,** we know that greed for the character Gordon Gekko didn't work out so well. However, the simple fact is that greed, if directed properly, can help us reach our goals.

I'm telling you right now, as I write these words — I am greedy for my former self. And, people can give us all the self-

---

affirmation, self-accepting crap they would like to dish out, but the simple truth is — none of us like being overweight and out of shape. Actually, the *love yourself the way you are* mantra can actually speed our demise. If we don't completely embrace that we desire to change, we never will.

I'm not saying we need to loathe or hate ourselves, far from it — yes we should love ourselves, but to say that we are better off being unfit, unhealthy and unwell because we choose not to take care of ourselves is not something that I desire — and if you are reading this book, obviously neither do you.

Do we desire to be healthier? Then let's be greedy for it.

Do we want to wear nice, well-fitting clothing? Then let's develop a hunger for it.

Do we want to be more attractive to our partner? Then let's crave it until we feel pangs in our bellies.

The need must be so strong that we hurt inside, and yet, we must know how much more we are hurting without that drive.

Replace the craving for food with a yearning to be fit. It is okay to be self-centered in our aspiration for vim and vigor -- it will take time, it will take discipline, it will take hard work for us to achieve our goals. We must allow ourselves the freedom to put us first while striving toward our goal. Just remember, never be selfish. When the work is done, we aren't doing this simply for ourselves.

We are doing it to be able to spend active, quality times with our loved ones. We are working toward not only feeling better, but being better, secure in the knowledge that we are now in control.

It will take some time to convince yourself that it is okay to be greedy for good health. We have been conditioned by religion, by family, by politicians and often times society as a whole, to put our own needs, wants and interests second. What we miss by living this way, is the fact that if we can't care for ourselves, how can we ever hope to care for others. An unfit, unhealthy body can lack the physical prowess to do the simplest tasks, let alone any heroic endeavor.

As the body becomes weak, the mind can follow. It is true that a fit body houses a healthy mind, so why are people so unwilling to accept the inverse? When we physically tire, our mental acuity declines, in the short term, this may require nothing more than a nap, but long term the effects can have health damaging repercussions.

To counteract the effects of an unfit body has on our brains, we drink way too much coffee, or worse, souped up energy drinks. For some reason, we are okay with putting off the long term consequences of bad habits, but we aren't willing to invest in the long term benefits of healthy habits.

If we feed our bodies good, solid, natural nutrients — the need for the overconsumption of caffeinated products will disappear.

If we devote the time and energy to physically condition our bodies, the fatigue that catches so many of us off guard, will become a rare occurrence.

By utilizing greed for good health, we can motivate ourselves to devote the time in making a better us — so not only us, but those we love, will enjoy a better life.

Stage 1: Denial

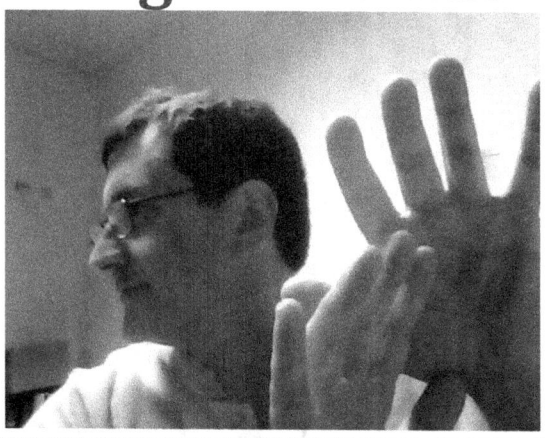

Boy did I go through this one, and this may have been my most difficult step to overcome. You see, I have a large frame, and when the weight starts to come on, it is very easy for me to dismiss it as putting on mass. Yes, fat is mass, but in my deluded brain, the mass was muscle. Even though my shirts weren't simply getting tighter in the shoulders, they were getting snug around the middle — but hey, when abs get bigger they push out; don't they?

I went through this stage for about three months. And, before I knew it, clothes were going from simply tight to no longer fitting, and workouts went from missing one or two, to only making one or two.

Stage 2: Anger

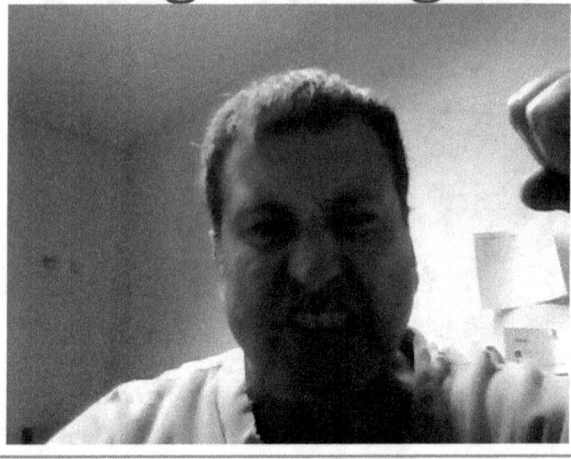

I talked about anger as a sin, but that doesn't mean it doesn't fit
here as well. In addition to the anger in my writing, I was
angry at myself. I must admit, I'm not sure I am 100% past
this stage. However, back when I entered this stage I was very
angry with myself. I would have long, heated conversations
with myself, asking, begging, demanding, *how could I let this
happen — again!* Now the anger is more centered on how I
could invest all that hard work into getting fit, only to let it slip
so easily. However, in time, the self-blame and internal anger
subsided into a honest self-assessment.

Stage 3: Bargaining

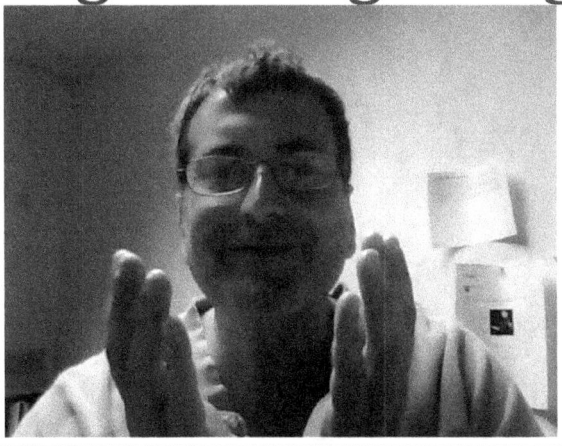

In this case bargaining is applied differently than in the stages of grief. This bargaining became more like — *Well, I can have this last ice cream cone today and tomorrow, I can get on track.* Or, *If I work out today, it won't be so bad if I miss tomorrow's workout.* This type of bargaining was self-destructive because, the bargain that had negative impacts on my health and fitness were "honored," while the healthier ends of the bargains always fell by the wayside.

Stage 4: Depression

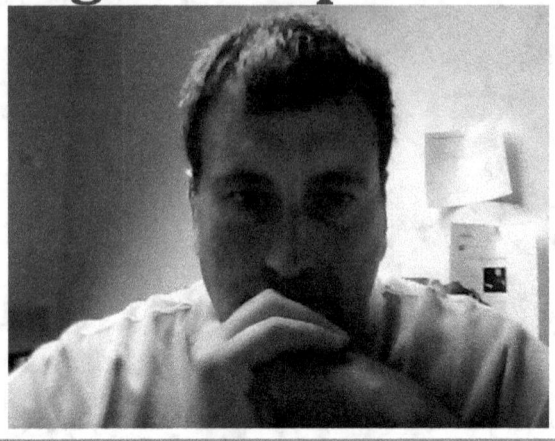

Not clinical depression, but an overt sadness became the dominant mood most of my days. This would evolve from the anger stage. The same issues I was angry about, now became the catalyst for sadness. Unfortunately, for carb-addicted people like myself, this stage ends up adding a significant amount of weight re-gain rapidly. I said this in Obesity Undone, and I will it say it here again, when depressed, food is the friend that is never too busy, the lover that never has a headache, and food always makes us feel the same way again and again. When we are sad or depressed, we desire comfort, and food, for better or worse; usually worse, has a way to transport us to times in our lives when we were children. Where, in my case, the smell of spaghetti sauce simmering on the stove brings back the security of being home with my mother or grandmother. The aroma transfers to the taste, and then the fullness of the belly has a way to magically make all the stressors, and the anxieties, and all the sadness just disappear — even if it is only momentarily. Thus, with larger problems — we become more hungry, not physically, but emotionally hungry for that comforted feeling. Therefore, we indulge over and over and over. As the numbers on the scale increase, as we switch to wearing larger sized clothing, the momentary comfort is replaced with even more sadness as we are realizing how out of control we are becoming. Thus, depression is not only an effect; it is also a cause.

Stage 5: Acceptance

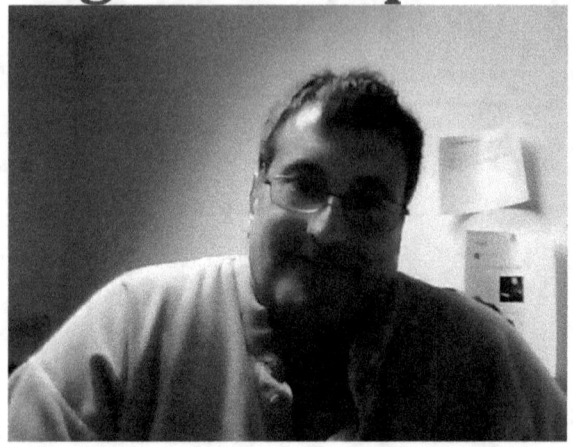

With acceptance, denial and bargaining are out of the picture, but components of depression and anger remain — and that isn't necessarily a bad thing. If harnessed the right way, that anger and sadness can be used as a catalyst to get back on track. In my case, I took to writing, which became the *"Important Week,"* blog postings, one which I reprinted earlier, and this posting, which unintentionally struck some nerves:

An Important Week — Honest Self-Assessment
July 25, 2013

"Then you will know the truth, and the truth will set you free." John 8.32

The most prominent theme in the comments I have received since I wrote An Important Week, have to do with me being too hard on myself. I must admit; this has me befuddled.

The words I chose, and continue choose, are to relay an honest assessment of where I was, where I had been and where I want to go. When we give ourselves open ended time frames, it is very easy to put off doing something until the next day, week, month or longer. I gave myself one week to get back on track — if I failed to do so, I was going to discontinue my public advocacy of living a healthier, more fit lifestyle. Really, if I continued championing fitness while weighing almost 300 pounds, and being out of shape, and doing nothing to remedy the situation — Who the hell would take me seriously? Perhaps more importantly — How could I take myself seriously?

I take the usage of language, either the spoken or written word, as an earnest expression of my inner thoughts. The words I use, whether they are positive and cheery, or not — are used to convey those ideas, not only to those who read what I wrote, but to myself as well.

I am often baffled at how we as a people proclaim how much we desire and respect honesty, yet, we don't like the use of words which are authentic. I failed myself for the last year — that is a plain, simple fact! I gained 84 pounds, and the endurance, strength and fitness I earned through hard work were all gone; what am I supposed to do — pat myself on the back? Should I tell myself — good job on gaining that weight back?

I remember growing up, it was admirable to display inner strength and mental toughness —Today, does everyone want their hand held?

I don't!

I screwed up!

And, here comes the other word people don't like to use — I was mentally WEAK! I ate, and ate, and ate, and ate. I consumed all of the foods I told others not to shove down their gullets. Instead of rising each day and tackling my waking hours with exercise, positive energy and gusto — I slept in. I sat around and drank coffee watching Mike and Mike In The Morning or Lead Off with Allie LaForce and Doug Gottlieb. Should I congratulate myself for watching reports of others being active and achieving?

This isn't about compassion, or lack thereof; it isn't about being nice, or not; it isn't about being sensitive or not?

Is it compassionate to lie to ourselves as our health deteriorates?

Is it nice to shower platitudes upon ourselves to the point that physical and mental fitness suffers?

Is it sensitive to stand by and simply watch behaviors that are self-destructive?

I think not!

At certain times it is important to not merely be candid — but to be brutally forthright. I was writing largely for myself. I am humbled that I inspire others; but I don't want that inspiration to be phony and hypocritical. If I can't face my weakness, if I can't accept that I failed, and most importantly, that I have the inner strength to overcome — how can I ever hope move others to do the same?

I could have easily hidden away, gotten back in shape, and most would not have been any the wiser. But then, I couldn't look myself in the mirror, I would not have been able to sleep at night and really, the only person who would have been fooled by such a ruse would have been me. I had to face the realities that I had let myself down — that I allowed my health to crumble. If I couldn't be authentic with myself — I could never be genuine with other people.

The opening quote may be considered cliché by some; but that doesn't make it untrue. Since I had the courage, grit and fortitude to be honest with myself — I am back on track and ready to not solely, and perhaps it is a blessing, once again undo obesity, but come out triumphant over recidivism.

This self-assessment went beyond simple acceptance, it went to the core of what caused my problem and that I needed to do something about it. I simply didn't verbalize my thoughts, I had them in written form. Once the words were on my screen, they were more than abstract thoughts, they were reality — a reality that I can now reinforce over and over again. Acceptance must be combined with complete honesty — if not, if we are not 100% genuine with ourselves, we are still in denial and we can never move forward.

Myth 1: Cut Calories To Lose Weight

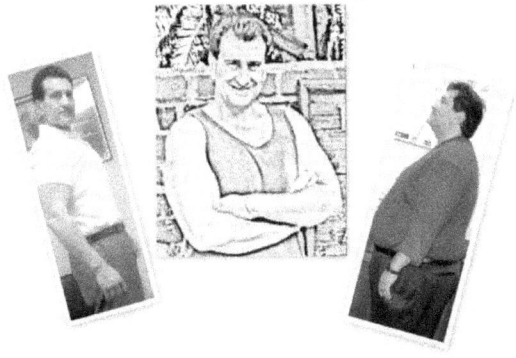

There are many out there that will tell you it is all about the calories, and there are just as many people who will tell you calories have nothing to do with it.

Which camp is correct? Both.

There is truth in each, just as there is misinformation as well.

I am a proponent of low carbohydrate eating. I didn't say no carb, I said low carb.

I don't count calories, and I don't 100% ascribe to the calories in/calories out model, however if I didn't give total caloric intake a passing consideration, I would be remiss. I'm not going to go over it again, I discussed it earlier in what I called the spare tank rule.

However, why low carb?

For me, it is a very personal consideration. Type II diabetes runs on both sides of my family, and while I am aware of arguments about what diet is best — I like to go with a common sense approach. More carbs equals more sugar equals more of a problem. If you want the science and physiology there are many places to find the information. If you want to hear some insightful interviews, visit my internet buddy Jimmy Moore's website. Jimmy has interviewed many of the top names in weight loss and fitness, including yours truly.

As many experts will argue about the best diet for type II diabetes, you will have just as many argue about whether dietary carbohydrates are even necessary. I don't really care if they are or aren't — the human body is smarter than any scientist, academic, researcher or clinician — we secrete enzymes to digest starches, so weather we require some dietary carbohydrate or not is irrelevant, our bodies can handle them and utilize them. In my case, and many others, too many carbohydrates cause us to gain weight, so we must be observant about the total amount we consume.

Whether or not carbohydrates are a necessary or a good energy source on the other hand, I say they are not. I would much rather burn fat for fuel any day. And, this is where the all calories are created equally goes out the window. The simple fact is that fats are much denser, 9kcal/gram compared to carbohydrates at 4kcal/gram. So, how the hell are carbohydrates a preferred source? They are not.

I always use a very simple example. I was born and raised in Northeastern Pennsylvania, also referred to as hard coal country. For decades, the coal mines here brought from the earth a harder type of coal known as anthracite, while coal from other regions is a soft coal called bituminous.

Anthracite is harder and more dense, thus it not only burns longer, but cleaner. Why? Because, like dietary fats, it is more energy dense. The more dense the fuel, the more effective the results.

As I have stated many times, I understand the science, physiology, etc... but sometimes we don't need much more than common sense to arrive at the best conclusion.

Myth 2: Reading Labels Is Important

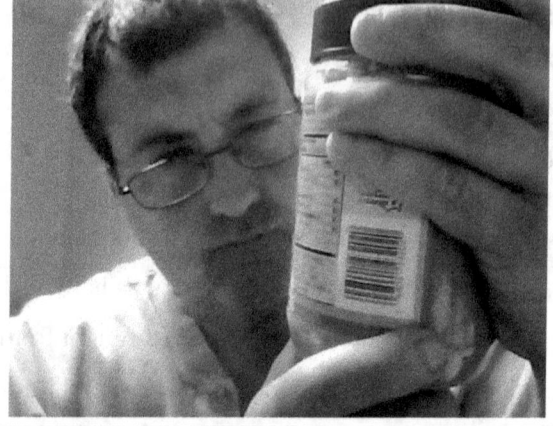

The short answer is — don't eat foods that have labels. The longer answer is — don't eat foods that have labels.

In my old YouTube postings, I always closed saying eat a diet low in carbohydrates and as close to nature as possible. As close to nature as possible doesn't require much in the way of labels. Jack LaLanne was fond of saying, shop the perimeter of a grocery store and avoid the aisles. If you follow that path, for the most part, you can't go wrong. Yes, there are some areas where there are packaged foods, but at this point, all we need to do is exercise common sense.

As we are losing weight, keep the foods to meats, poultry, seafood and vegetables. Use butter, coconut oil or lard for cooking, and olive oil and vinegar for dressing. Can we be perfect all the time? Of course not. But just by eating as close to nature as possible, we can rarely go wrong.

When it comes to eating out, and with my schedule, that can happen quite a bit, when in a pinch we can eat low carb fast foods. Most places have some type of salad variety, unsweetened iced tea, and when we need to — simply grab a burger or grilled chicken sandwich and toss the bun aside.

I have tried to make this chapter a little longer, but there really isn't much else to say. The best piece of advice is don't purchase food that requires labeling, therefore you won't have to worry about understanding those long words that belong more in the packaging than the food.

Myth 3: Don't Lose Weight Too Quickly

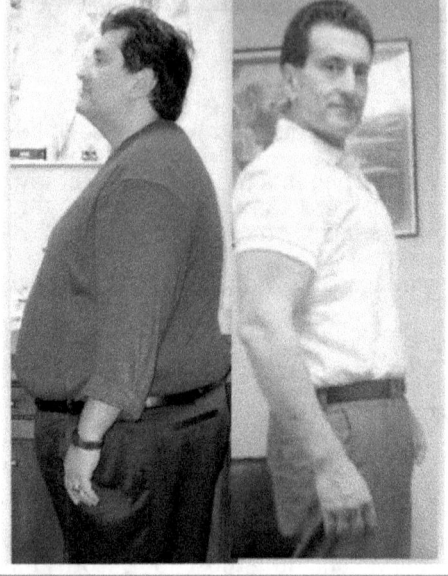

When someone says to me, *They say you shouldn't lose weight to quickly*, I usually give a 2 word answer — Bite Me!

I know — immature, but I simply can't help myself. The photos at the top of this section were taken exactly 1 year to the day apart, after a weight loss of 140 pounds. Was that too quick? Hell, I don't think it was quick enough. But, I never worry about how fast the weight comes off, it simply comes off as it comes off. Except for a period of time I was bulking up to compete in a strong man contest, I maintained a weight of about 210 pounds for about 3 ½ years.

Who deems how fast is too fast? You got me, I eat what I eat every day. I do my exercise routine every day. I try to keep a positive mental energy level every day. If I drop 3 pounds one week, and 7 the next and then no weight the following — I don't worry about it. I just keep working to make progress forward.

Too quickly? I never hear anyone use that lame ass statement in other aspects of life.

Can you imagine the stupidity. "*Wow, dude, Mr. Steve Jobs. It is like really cool to meet ya.* **(I know he's dead, just go with it)** *I admire you dude, but one thing. Man, I think you became a millionaire way too fast. I'm going to build a world class technology company, but I want to do it the right way, so I am going to spend like 40 years doing it.*"

Or

"LeBron James, you are such an incredible basketball player. One day I want to be just as good as you, but instead of making it to the NBA when I'm 18 years old, I want to wait until I'm 38. You know, I don't want to do it too quickly."

Myth 4: Use Food As A Reward

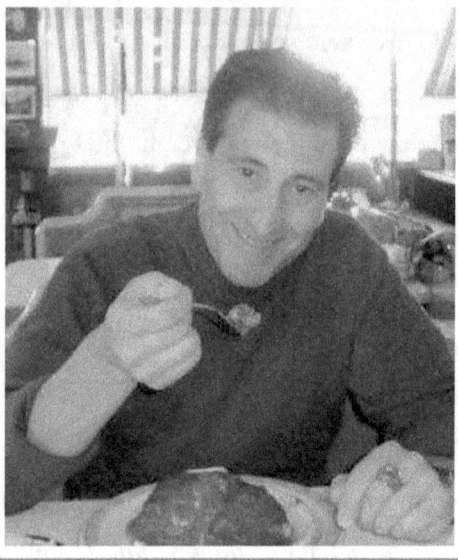

Now, here is a topic that I have kind of changed my mind a bit on. While in my first book, I never specifically use food as a reward, I do not only accept, but I encourage what the one and only Jimmy Moore termed *"planned splurges."* I never called them a reward, but some people had misinterpreted what my meaning was, so I will take a moment to make my point clear here.

I still think it is okay to have a planned splurge, in which you eat a favorite food or two, that you may not normally eat, one day every month or so. I used to advocate doing these splurges about once every two weeks, but many people told me they had difficulty getting back on track, so I changed it to monthly. After this bout of recidivism, I may make it even less. I'm not sure if I could be as disciplined as Jack LaLanne to never eat sweets again, but who knows, it is a goal for which I may strive.

The thing about these planned splurges that makes them different than a reward, is the word reward. The splurges weren't a reward for being good, they were actually worked into my lifestyle. By planning ahead, we have the ability to not get too sidetracked. The important thing about these splurges, if you choose indulge, is that it is one meal.

Let me repeat that — one meal.

Not one day, not a weekend, not on a vacation. It is a one meal splurge.

What happens in the reward model, is that the food becomes an entitlement, and that entitlement, like many government entitlements, can grow out of control. If we go, from one meal to two, to three to days to weeks, we are no longer eating healthy, we are back to eating a poor diet, and that simply isn't the goal of living a fit and healthy lifestyle.

Myth 5: You Require Carbs To Be Athletic

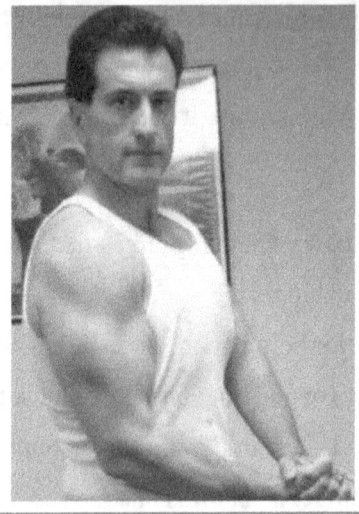

The above picture is from 2009 when I dropped my weight down from 340lbs… I reached that goal on a low carb diet of about 20-30 grams per day. After this bout of recidivism, and 4 years older, do I think I can do it again? You bet your ass.

I didn't need large amounts of carbohydrates then, I don't need them now. Currently, I am jogging roughly 2 miles a day, on certain days I do sprints and skip rope after my jog, and I lift weights 6 days a week. I have no problem with energy or strength or endurance.

Prevent The Cycle
Use The Scale

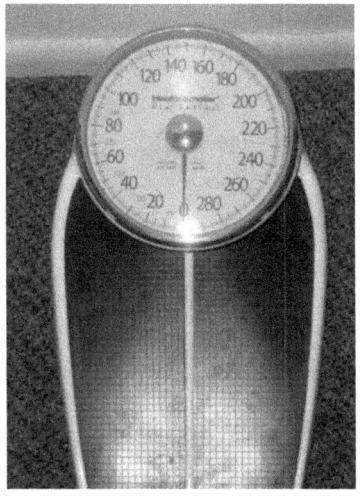

It is the friend we love to hate.

It is the teller of the truth.

It tells us no lies.

It is — the scale.

Look at the picture. It is an unassuming device. Nothing more than a platform over a spring, a dial covered by glass and a pointer connected to the spring. The digital variety are a little different, as is the physician's beam model. However, they are still pretty much all the same — they give us feedback.

The scale doesn't mean us any harm.

The scale doesn't mean to upset us.

The scale doesn't mean anger us.

Those of us who battle obesity, both love and despise the innocent little scale. As the weight is falling off, and it confirms the fruits of our labor, we celebrate it. However, when the reading is not so positive, if it doesn't move down, or worse, it moves up ever so slightly — we curse it.

Unfortunately, many become slaves to the scale, their very mood for the day is based upon the tale the pointer tells. That shouldn't be. The scale is a tool, nothing more and nothing less. It is an important tool, because not only does it track our progress, or lack thereof — it is a instrument of accountability. This purpose, should be its primary role.

As I wrote about in Obesity Undone, I advocate daily weighing, not to mark progress, but to maintain accountability, and during this bout of recidivism, I strayed from the scale. When I wasn't being good, I told myself — *I just need a couple of days to get on track, this way the reading won't be so bad.*

Sadly, I couldn't string together those couple of days, and avoidance became the norm.

It becomes self-defeating. We don't hop on the dreaded, dammed device, because we don't want to see what it will tell us — the truth.

The longer we avoid, the more difficult it becomes to get back on. We ignore other signs, the tightness of the clothes, we rationalize, that they must have shrunk in the wash. The mirror, suddenly only reflects us from the neck up. And the additional effort to heft our bulk from a chair — well, that's just old age.

We must take our heads from the sand, remove the blinders and accept the truth the scale tells. Or, like what happened to me, one day it will read 294.

During this relapse, I am often asked what my goals are for weight loss. Those of you who have been following my blog and YouTube channel are aware my focus is primarily on improving overall fitness levels. However, yes I want to drop weight, but improving my health is the overriding desire. Body weight, body fat, clothing size and body habitus are tools utilized in monitoring that improvement.

I do have a goal weight; it may change the closer I get to it, depending on how I feel, how clothing fits, etc… I use the target weight to assist me in achieving my overall intention.

The next question I usually get asked is "When do you want to reach that goal?" My answer is always the same,

"Whenever I get there."

I receive many other questions, but for the most part, people don't believe that I don't have a set date by which to lose weight. I further explain that having a set date is pointless, because my overall goal isn't simply the number on the scale. However, I elaborate, clarifying that when people set a date or an event, to reach their goal, what usually occurs is a letdown, sometimes brief, other times so bad that it leads to rebounding and recidivism.

I have also been accused of losing weight too fast at certain times. I give a perplexed look and then I ask a simple question, "Why?" The answer back is always the same, "Because they say you shouldn't lose weight too fast." If you have read either edition of my book, you will know how I feel about them, but I won't go there today.

Simply put, I do nothing drastically differently when I am dropping weight compared to when I am maintaining. I don't starve myself, I don't sit endlessly in a sauna and I don't work out much differently. I eat my meals, which usually are between four and six feedings a day, I jog, skip rope, do sprints and lift weights in some combination every day, regardless of my body weight. The only slight alteration in my diet is that I add back in some fruit as I near my target weight, and when I am maintaining, I add a little additional fruit and some naturally occurring, unprocessed starches like a sweet potato or yam. The only changes in my exercise may be a little more distance, heavier weights and quicker and longer sessions — but that is simply because I am in better physical condition, it is part of the process of getting in shape, once you're there, the body adapts by being able to do more work.

Since the overall objective is improved fitness, to improve health, to live a better life — we mustn't get wrapped up on a set date or some event — get focused on a lifetime change and remember weight loss is a side effect of fitness; fitness is not the end result of weight loss.

What Do We Do Now?

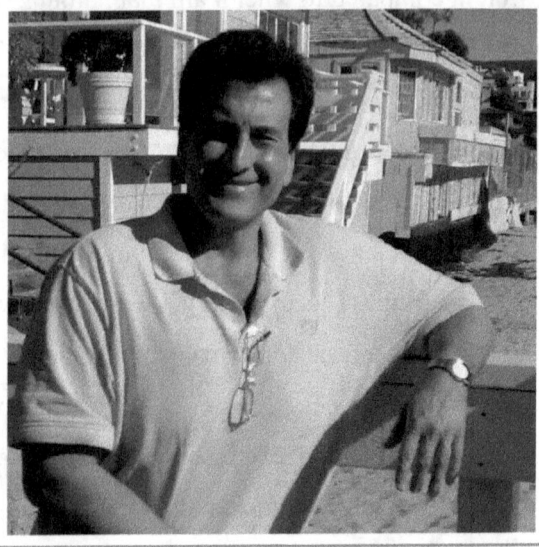

First we smile. We take a moment to be thankful for all the good we have in life; even if it isn't much, find it and hold on to it. This is where we will build from and upon.

Next, we stop feeling sorry for ourselves and we stop eating crap, and we get off of our asses and start exercising. Some of my life downright sucks. Financially, I haven't recovered from the misdiagnosis that took me out of my practice for several months back in 2006 — that is 7 years at the time of this writing. I spent a lot of time blaming other people, but the simple truth is that I responded poorly, and those poor responses, and my decisions have slowed my financial recovery.

Yet, I have so much good in life, so much for which to be thankful. I love my practice, teaching, being a business person and doing physical culture. And, most of all, I have a great family and friends.

My girlfriend, her daughter, my sisters and nephews are all so important to me. I want to be healthy and fit to enjoy my time with them. We get one ride on this trip called life, how we spend it in large part depends not on the good luck or the adversity, but how we respond to what is thrown at us.

Besides eating and exercise, our mental energy is our dearest friend. We must strive to be positive each and every day. We must block out the negative influences that surround us, that try to engulf us, we must be stronger than our weakest moments.

Most importantly, after we isolate what has brought us to this place, after we have been earnest and honest, we must forgive ourselves and move forward. It is one thing to identify the issue, but it is quite another to dwell on it.

Recognizing what caused either our initial obesity or recidivism is important and healthy, dwelling on it, beating ourselves up eternally, will only lead us back down the path of an unhealthy, unfit and unfruitful life — we do what we do for just the opposite reason — to live a better life.

Also, we can take comfort in the fact that it isn't all that complicated. Life is lived in color, but sometimes the answers remain black and white.

Aloha, Ciao, and Stay Healthy,

Joe

If you want my eating, exercise, and energy information it is in my book Obesity Undone, paperback or kindle version, or on my website ObesityUndone.com.

Epilogue:
Recidivism Undone

Below are photos chronicling my battle back over the bastard that is obesity.

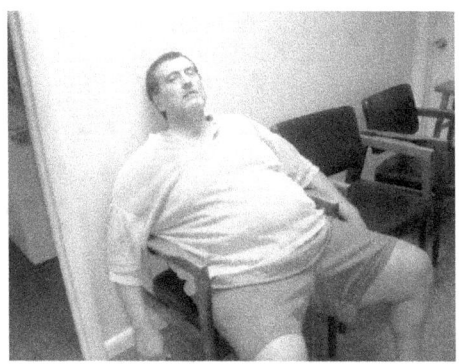

7/26/13 294 pounds

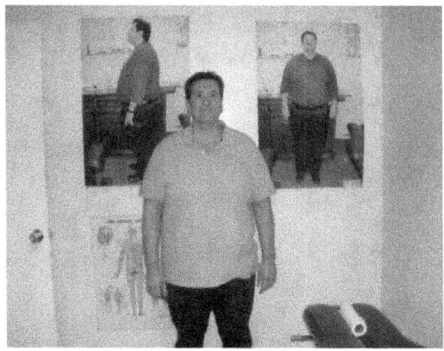

9/18/13 269 pounds 25 pounds gone

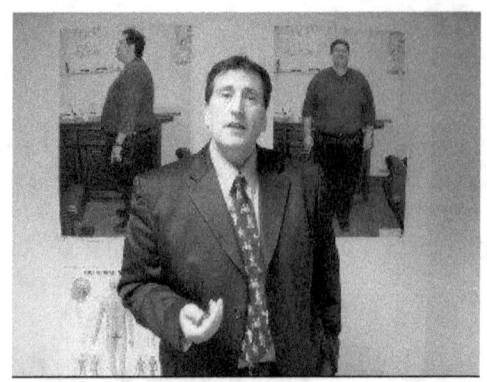

10/31/13 252 pounds ½ way point

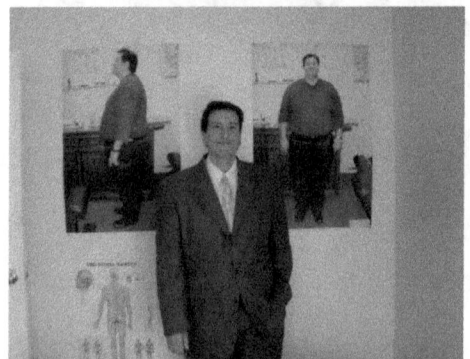

11/13/13 244 pounds 50 pounds gone

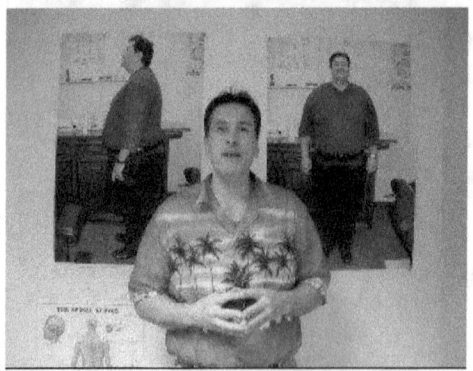

12/23/13 235 pounds 25 pounds to go

www.ingramcontent.com/pod-product-compliance
Lightning Source LLC
Chambersburg PA
CBHW072250310526
45795CB00011B/631